MEDIASTINAL TUMORS

IN

CHILDHOOD

A dissertation

Submitted to the scientific council of thoracic and cardiovascular surgery in partial fulfillment of the requirement for the degree of fellowship of the Iraqi board for medical specializations.2012

By

Saif Sami Al-mudhaffar

M.B.Ch.B

Supervised by

Professor

Emad AL-Mashat

F.R.C.S. F.L.L.U.M.C.

Chairman of the scientific

Council of Thoracic and

Cardiovascular surgery

Summary

Aim of study:

Mediastinal tumors in children comprise a heterogeneous group of lesions that have a range of embryonic origins. They may present as benign cysts, as well as malignant lesions. this study was planned to describe the diagnostic procedures, the treatments and outcomes of a group of children and adolescents with mediastinal tumors.

Methods:

A retrospective analysis of 35 children with mediastinal tumors who were treated at medical city Thoracic and Vascular surgery department, from January 2009 to December 2010. All patients were submitted to some kind of surgical procedure: diagnostic, therapeutic, or both.

Results:

Out of the (35) patients who were studied, there were 6 (19%) female and 29 (81%) male patients in the study. The patients ranged in age from 14 days to 15 years at the time of diagnosis, with a mean age of (8.4) years. Histological confirmation was made in all patients.

Conclusion:

The most common tumors in the anterior mediastinum were lymphomas. In posterior mediastinum the most common were neurogenic tumors. Surgery is an important step for the diagnosis and treatment of such lesions.

Chapter one

1.1   Introduction

The mediastinum is defined as that space that lies between the two pleural cavities. Within this space lie many vital structures. Superiorly the mediastinum is bordered by the thoracic inlet; and inferiorly it is bordered by the thoracic surface of the diaphragm. The sternum comprises the anterior border while the spine comprises the posterior border. Traditionally, the mediastinum has been divided into three imaginary compartments: anterior, middle (or visceral), and posterior. Although such a division is convenient from an anatomical and surgical standpoint, it should be noted that structures located predominantly in one compartment may encroach upon, or involve, another compartment. For instance, the thymus, located in the anterior mediastinum, may extend into the middle mediastinum in certain pathological states[1].

1.2 MEDIASTINAL ANATOMY

The most classic description as described in Gray's Anatomy[2] divides the mediastinum into four compartments: superior, anterior, middle, and posterior. The superior mediastinum includes all structures from the thoracic inlet superiorly to a line drawn from the lower edge of the manubrium to the lower edge of the fourth thoracic vertebrae, inferiorly. Inferior to this line is the inferior mediastinum, which is subsequently divided into three parts anterior, middle, and posterior compartments that are bounded inferiorly by the diaphragm. The boundary between the anterior and middle compartments is the anterior pericardium; between the middle and posterior compartments is the posterior aspect of the tracheal bifurcation, pulmonary vessels, and pericardium. A revision of the four-compartment system combines the anterior and superior compartments into an anterosuperior compartment, thus creating three compartments[3] . (Fig. 1)

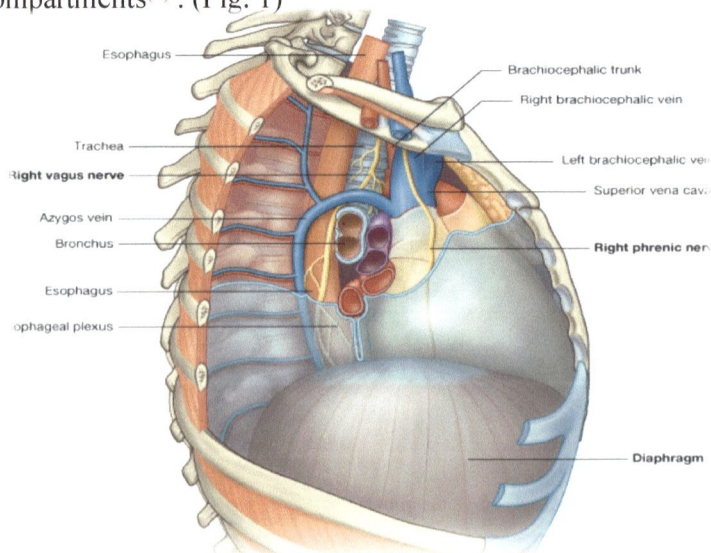

Fig. 1: Mediastinal Anatomy (grays' anatomy –chapter 3) [4]

An alternative model proposed by Shields in 1972[3] is perhaps the most straight forward . This describes a three-compartment model consisting of an anterior compartment, middle (or visceral) compartment, and a posterior compartment (paraventral sulcus). All three compartments are bounded inferiorly by the diaphragm, laterally by the pleural space, and superiorly by the thoracic inlet. The anterior compartment is bounded anteriorly by the sternum and posteriorly by the great vessels and pericardium. It contains the thymus, internal mammary vessels, fat, connective tissue, and potentially structures such as ectopic parathyroid tissue or a substernal goiter. Dorsal to the anterior compartment is the visceral compartment or middle mediastinum, which is bounded posteriorly by the ventral surface of the thoracic spine. The visceral compartment occupies the entire thoracic inlet and contains the great vessels, heart, pericardium, trachea, proximal mainstem bronchi, vagus nerves, phrenic nerves, esophagus, thoracic duct, descending aorta, and azygous venous system. The posterior compartment of the mediastinum or paraventral sulcus consists of potential spaces along the thoracic vertebrae that contain the sympathetic chain, proximal portions of the intercostal neurovascular bundles, thoracic spinal ganglia, and the distal azygous vein (Fig. 2). The paraventral sulci are not technically in the mediastinum but contain structures that give rise to pathology that is classically considered in the posterior mediastinum (neurogenic tumors)[3].

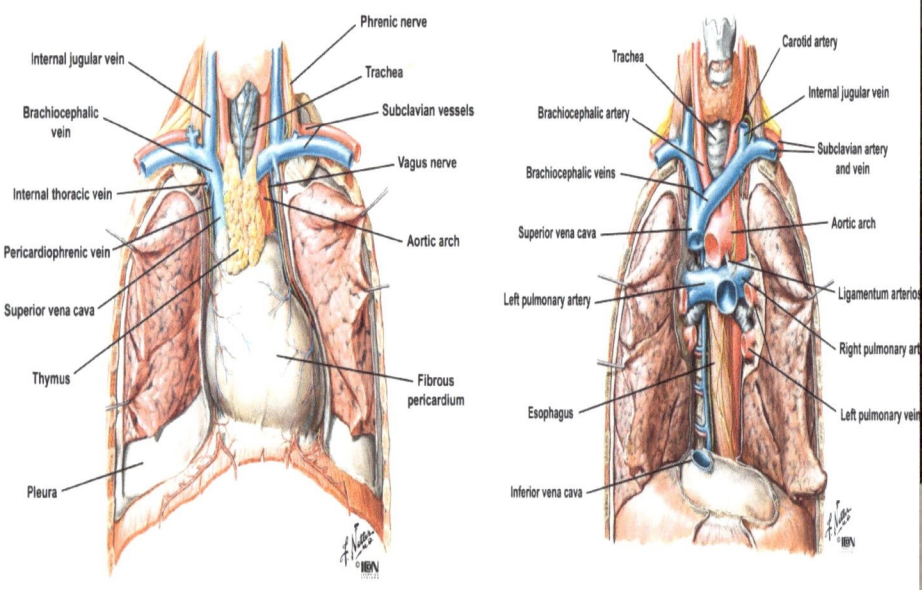

(a)   (b)

Fig.2 : Content of mediastinum :

   (a) : Anterior mediastinum

   (b) : Middle (visceral) mediastinum

1.3   POTENTIAL SPACES IN THE MEDIASTINUM

When mediastinal anatomy is discussed, several potential spaces are described, most often in conjunction with staging lung cancer. The pretracheal space is a triangular space bounded anterolaterally by the superior vena cava and right brachiocephalic vein on the right, the aorta and pericardium on the left, and posteriorly by the trachea. This is the space explored by standard mediastinoscopy and is continous inferiorly with the subcarinal space. The subcarinal space is bounded superiorly by the carina, laterally by the mainstem bronchi, anteriorly by the pulmonary artery, and posteriorly by the esophagus   . The aortopulmonary window is the space bounded superiorly by the aortic arch, medially by the trachea and esophagus, inferiorly by the pulmonary artery, and laterally by the pleura. This space contains lymph nodes, the ligamentum arteriosum, and the left recurrent laryngeal nerve and can be accessed by an anterior mediastinotomy, extended cervical mediastinoscopy, or thoracoscopy/thoracotomy, [5].as shown in Fig.3.

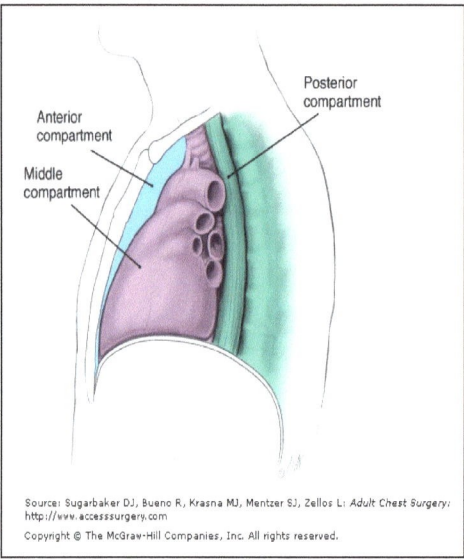
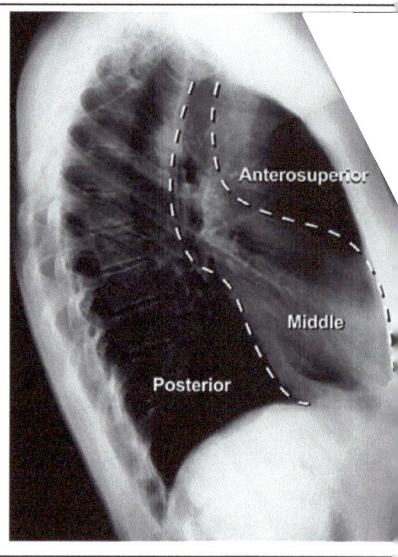

Fig.3: Compartements of mediastinum.

1.4 MEDIASTINAL LYMPH NODE ANATOMY

In 1997 the American Joint Committee and the Union Internationale Contre le Cancer adopted a regional lymph node classification in order to unify two previously utilized systems and provide a consistent, reproducible means of classifying thoracic lymph nodes.[5] This system, used primarily for staging lung cancer, classifies lymph nodes into 14 different stations based on anatomical position. Node stations 1 through 9 are contained within the mediastinal pleura and thus are mediastinal lymph nodes. Lymph node stations 2, 4, and 7 are depicted in and are the only nodal stations accessible by standard mediastinoscopy. Lymph node stations 5 and 6 are depicted in and are not accessible by routine mediastinoscopy, (Fig. 4) [5]

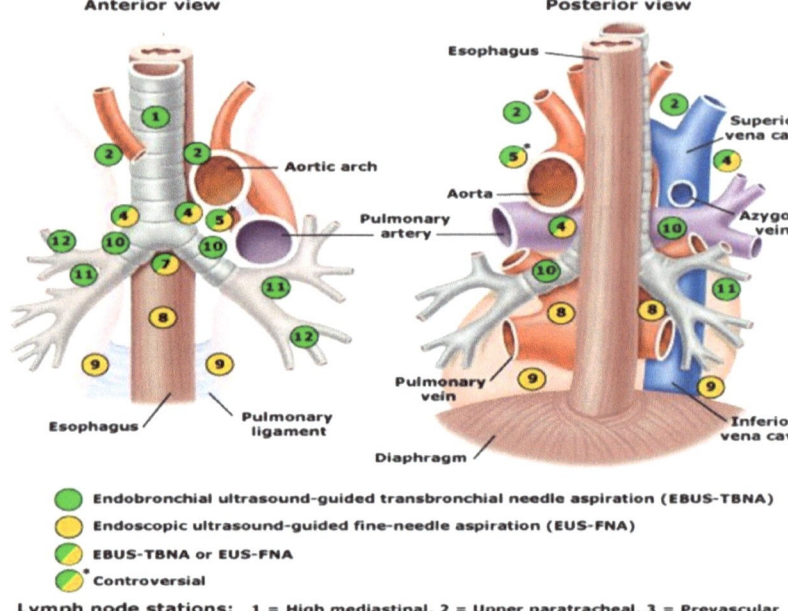

Fig.4:

Anterior view

Posterior view

Esophagus

Aortic arch

Aorta

Pulmonary artery

Superior vena cav

Azygou vein

Esophagus

Pulmonary ligament

Pulmonary vein

Inferior vena cav

Diaphragm

● Endobronchial ultrasound-guided transbronchial needle aspiration (EBUS-TBNA)

◐ Endoscopic ultrasound-guided fine-needle aspiration (EUS-FNA)

◐ EBUS-TBNA or EUS-FNA

◐* Controversial

Lymph node stations: 1 = High mediastinal, 2 = Upper paratracheal, 3 = Prevascular and retrotracheal (not shown), 4 = Lower paratracheal, 5 = Aortopulmonary window, 6 = Para-aortic (not shown), 7 = Subcarinal, 8 = Paraesophageal, 9 = Pulmonary ligament, 10 = Hilar, 11 = Interlobar, 12 = Lobar

1.5   Etiology and Embryology

In addition to classification by location, mediastinal masses can also be categorized as developmental, neoplastic, or inflammatory. It is presumed that incomplete separation and tubulization of the esophagus and trachea after the proliferative phase, which normally occurs by the fifth week of gestation, results in foregut duplication. Additionally, these duplication cysts can communicate with the spinal canal, and are referred to as neuroenteric cysts. The thymus develops as paired primordium from the ventral third pharyngeal pouch and descends to an area anterior to the aortic arch during the seventh week of gestation. Incomplete descent or obliteration of its tract may result in a cystic or ectopic thymus in the neck. In the middle mediastinum, bronchogenic cysts develop from abnormal budding of the tracheal diverticulum or ventral portion of the foregut. Pericardial cysts occur from the failure of disconnected lacunae in the mesenchyme to coalesce to form the pericardial sac. [6]

The most common neoplasm of the anterior mediastinum in children is lymphoma, accounting for up to 45% of pediatric mediastinal masses. Germ cell tumors (25%), mesenchymal tumors (15%), and thymic tumors (17%) comprise the remainder. Most of these tumors are malignant. Neurogenic lesions, which comprise approximately 20% of mediastinal tumors, are usually located in the posterior mediastinum. Many developmental conditions of the mediastinum (i.e., thymic cysts, enteric cysts, bronchogenic cysts, and cystic hygroma) are at increased risk for acquired infection[7].

Most mediastinal masses are asymptomatic, but many can be associated with specific symptoms and signs. Symptoms depend on the size of the lesion, whether it is benign or malignant, and the presence or absence of infection. It is generally agreed that malignant lesions are more likely to be symptomatic than benign lesions. Approximately 25% of all mediastinal tumors are malignant in both adults and children. Roughly two-thirds of children are symptomatic at presentation. Most symptoms are related to mediastinal structures that have been either compressed or invaded by tumor. These consist of respiratory symptoms such as cough, stridor, hemoptysis, and Dyspnea or pain related to invasion of the chest wall, mediastinal pleura, or diaphragm. Other symptoms and signs may include dysphagia, hoarseness, superior vena cava syndrome , pericardial tamponade, Horner's syndrome, and reticular pain owing to extension into vertebral foramina[8].

1.6   Clinical Presentation

Most mediastinal masses are often discovered incidentally on chest Radiographs taken for other indications. However, clinical symptoms are frequently the result of mass effects on normal structures within a particular compartment. Large masses in the anterior and middle mediastinum are particularly significant for their potential influence on respiratory tract symptoms, including airway obstruction.

Symptoms may range from noisy stridorous breathing in infants, to cough, chest pain, Dyspnea, and orthopnea in older children [9]. Cardiac compression may result in cyanosis, syncope, and dysrhythmias. Great vessel compression can lead to superior vena cava syndrome, characterized by venous engorgement along with head and neck swelling. By contrast, posterior mediastinal masses can be quite large and yet remains asymptomatic. However, posterior mediastinal masses, especially those that enter neural foramina, can cause symptoms of spinal cord compression. Certain pathology presents with specific symptoms. Hodgkin's lymphomas may have concomitant cervical or supraclavicular nodes as well as fever, night sweats and weight loss ('B' symptoms) in one-third of patients. Neuroblastoma in the upper mediastinum involving the stellate ganglion produces Horner's syndrome, characterized by ptosis, miosis, and anhydrosis. Although rare, a pediatric patient with thymic neoplasia may present with myasthenia gravis or hypoplastic anemia.[10]

Symptoms related to compression or invasion of mediastinal structures, such as the superior vena caval syndrome, Horner's syndrome, hoarseness, and severe pain, are more indicative of a malignant histologic diagnosis, although patients with a benign lesion, on occasion, present in this manner.

A number of primary mediastinal lesions produce hormones or antibodies that cause systemic symptoms, which may characterize a specific syndrome. Examples of these syndromes include Cushing's syndrome, caused by ectopic production of adrenocorticotropic hormone, most frequently by neuroendocrine tumors; thyrotoxicosis, caused by a mediastinal goiter; hypertension and a hyperdynamic state, caused by pheochromocytoma; and hypercalcemia secondary to increased parathyroid hormone release from a mediastinal parathyroid adenoma table (1).[11]

Table (1): Systemic Syndromes Caused by Mediastinal Neoplasm Hormone Production

SYNDROME	TUMOR
Hypertension	Pheochromocytoma, chemodectoma, ganglioneuroma, neuroblastoma
Hypoglycemia	Mesothelioma, teratoma, fibrosarcoma, neurosarcoma
Diarrhea	Ganglioneuroma, neuroblastoma, Neurofibroma
Hypercalcemia	Parathyroid adenoma/carcinoma, Hodgkin's disease
Thyrotoxicosis	Thyroid adenoma/carcinoma
Gynecomastia	Nonseminomatous germ cell tumor

Mediastinal masses are most frequently located in the anterosuperior mediastinum (54%), with the posterior (26%) and middle mediastinum (20%) being less frequently involved.[1] Many of the mediastinal lesions occur in characteristic sites within the mediastinum. The masses that occur most commonly in each of the three anatomic subdivisions are shown in Table (2) . In addition, the location of the mass explains some of the typical symptoms related to a mediastinal mass because of compression or invasion of adjacent mediastinal structures. (11)

Table (2) : Differential Diagnosis of Mediastinal Tumors by Location

Anterosuperior Mediastinum

95% of tumors in this compartment made up by the four "Ts":
    Thymoma
    Teratoma (germ cell tumors)
    Thyroid goiter
    "Terrible" lymphoma

Middle Mediastinum

Majority are cysts
    Most common: congenital foregut cysts (20% of all mediastinal masses)
    Bronchogenic cysts
    Pericardial cysts

Most common tumor in middle mediastinum:
    Lymphoma

Posterior Mediastinum

Neurogenic
    Nerve sheath subtype
        Benign
        Malignant
    Paraganglionic subtype
        Benign

Malignant

1.7   PRIMARY NEOPLASMS

Mediastinal tumors and cysts affect people of all ages, although they are more common in young and middle-aged adults. Most mediastinal masses are diagnosed in an asymptomatic patient on routine chest radiographs. Symptoms may occur as a result of local involvement of adjacent structures, tumor secretory factors, or immunologic factors. Benign lesions are more commonly asymptomatic, whereas malignant lesions generally produce clinical findings. The precise nature of a mediastinal lesion is dependent on histology. However, a tentative preoperative diagnosis can often be made by consideration of location of the tumor, age of the patient, presence or absence of local symptoms, and association of a specific systemic disease state[12]. With improvements in treatment modalities, the observation of a mediastinal mass, except in rare circumstances, cannot be justified. Although differences in the relative incidence of neoplasms and cysts exist in some series, the most common mediastinal masses are neurogenic tumors (23%), thymomas (21%), lymphomas (13%) and germ cell tumors (12%).

Table (3): Classification of Primary Mediastinal Tumors and Cysts[12]

BENIGN	MALIGNANT
Thymic	
Hyperplasia	**Invasive thymoma**
Thymic cysts	**Thymic carcinoma**
Encapsulated thymoma	**Thymic neuroendocri**
Thymolipoma	**Thymic lymphoma**
Germ cell tumors	
Mature teratoma	**Immature teratoma**
Immature teratoma (age <15)	**Teratoma with malig transformation**
Mature teratoma with immature elements <50% of the tumor volume	**Seminoma**

	Nonseminomatous ge tumors
	Mixed germ cell tum
Endocrine tumors	
Multinodularsubsternal goiter	**Substernal thyroid c**
Substernal thyroid	
Parathyroid substernal adenomas	
Parathyroid substernal cysts	
Lymph node masses	
Infectious hyperplasia	**Lymphoma**
Sarcoid hyperplasia of lymph nodes	**Metastatic lymphatic enlargement**
Castleman's disease	
Mesenchymal tumors	
Lipomatosis	**Liposarcoma**
Lipoma	
Fibroma	
Hemangioma	**Angiosarcoma**
Hemangioendothelioma	
Hemangiopericytoma	**Malignant hemangio**
Lymphangioma	**Lymphangiosarcoma**
Cystic hygroma	
Mediastinallymphangioma	**Lymphangiopericyto**
Lymphangiomatosis	
Cysts	
Bronchogenic	
Pericardial	
Esophageal duplication cysts	
Mesothelial cysts	

The incidence of mediastinal masses varies in infants, children, and adultsThe neurogenic tumors in children most commonly originate from sympathetic ganglion cells: gangliomas, ganglioneuroblastomas, and neuroblastomas. In contrast, neurilemomas and neurofibromas are the most common neurogenic tumors in adults. The childhood lymphomas are usually of a non-Hodgkin's lymphoma variety. The germ cell tumors are most frequently benign teratomas. Pericardial cysts and thymomas are uncommon in children[12].

Clinical Manifestations of Anatomic Compression or Invasion by Neoplasm's of the Mediastinum[11]

Spinal cord compressive syndrome
Vena caval obstruction
Pericardial tamponade
Congestive heart failure
Dysrhythmias
Pulmonary stenosis
Tracheal compression
Esophageal compression
Vocal cord paralysis
Horner's syndrome
Phrenic nerve paralysis
Chylothorax
Chylopericardium
Pancoast's syndrome
Postobstructive pneumonitis

1.8   Diagnosis

The goal of the diagnostic evaluation in a patient with a mediastinal mass is a precise histologic diagnosis so that optimal therapy can be performed. The preoperative evaluation of a patient with a mediastinal mass is intended to achieve the following[12]:

1. Differentiate a primary mediastinal mass from masses of other causes that have a similar radiographic appearance
2. Recognize associated systemic manifestations that may affect the patient's perioperative course
3. Evaluate for possible compression by the mass of the tracheobronchial tree, pulmonary artery, or superior vena cava
4. Ascertain whether the mass extends into the spinal column
5. Determine whether the mass is a nonseminomatous germ cell tumor
6. Assess the likelihood of respectability
7. Identify significant factors of medical comorbidity and optimize overall medical condition

The initial diagnostic intervention needs to be a careful history and physical examination.

 The recognition of associated systemic syndromes with many neoplasms is necessary to avoid potentially serious intraoperative and postoperative complications. Although most systemic syndromes are of little consequence regarding the planned surgical management, the association of myasthenia gravis, malignant hypertension, hypogammaglobulinemia, hypercalcemia, and thyrotoxicosis with mediastinal neoplasms markedly affects appropriate management.

Investigations Modalities include the followings:

1. The posteroanterior and lateral chest radiographs provide important information concerning anatomic location and size of the tumor.
2. Chest computed Tomography (CT) and magnetic resonance imaging (MRI) allows for determination of location, size, shape, density and composition of the mass, calcification, edge characteristics, lymphadenopathy, and associated findings. Considerable information can be obtained regarding the relative invasiveness and malignant nature of the mediastinal mass with either CT or MRI. Tumor disruption of fat planes; irregularity of pleural, vascular, or

pericardial margins by tumor; and infiltration into muscle or periosteum are useful for differentiating tumor compression from invasion. Resectability is better assessed than nonresectability using CT or MRI. MRI may be more useful than CT with certain posterior mediastinal masses in terms of evaluating foramen involvement in neurogenic tumors, and it has been shown to be superior to CT in diagnosing various cysts. Additionally, MRI may provide information regarding the involvement of the tumor with major vascular or cardiac structures and may help detect whether the tumor is actually a vascular abnormality[13].

3. Echocardiography may be useful in the evaluation of mediastinal masses, especially tumors that occur in the middle mediastinum or in patients with tamponade or pulmonary stenosis. Echocardiography delineates the cystic nature of lesions, and it has been used to guide needle biopsy, especially with lesions adjacent to the chest wall. Although echocardiography is not as sensitive as MRI or CT, it is useful in determining the physiologic effect of tumor involvement of the pericardium, heart, or great vessels.

4. Positron emission tomography (PET) and FDG (2-deoxy-2-[^{18}F] fluoro-d-glucose) has played an

increasing role in evaluation of mediastinal neoplasms, especially in determining the malignant potential of a mediastinal mass. One series reported the sensitivity and specificity of CT and PET in diagnosing tumor invasion and found PET to be superior (sensitivity, 90%; specificity, 92%; accuracy, 91%), while CT (sensitivity, 70%; specificity, 83%; accuracy, 77%). With thymic neoplasms, high FDG uptake was reflective of invasiveness and was seen in thymic carcinomas and invasive thymomas.[13] FDG-PET has a significantly higher sensitivity compared with gallium-67 (^{67}Ga) scintigraphy in pretherapy imaging of aggressive non-Hodgkin's lymphomas and Hodgkin's disease.[14]

5. Serologic evaluation is indicated in certain patients. Male patients in their second through fifth decades who have an anterosuperiormediastinal mass need to have α-fetoprotein and β-human chorionic gonadotropin (β-HCG) serologic studies obtained. A positive serology is indicative of a nonseminomatous germ cell tumor[14].

6. Urinary vanillylmandelic acid and catecholamines measurement. Is indicated in patients with mediastinal mass Patients with a mediastinal mass and a history hypertension or hypermetabolism. This enables the initiation of appropriate preoperative adrenergic blockers in patients with hormonally active intrathoracic

pheochromocytoma, paraganglioma, and neuroblastoma, limiting preoperative complications secondary to episodic catecholamine release. In these patients, nuclear scans using metaiodobenzylguanidine (MIBG) are useful in tumor location and in identifying sites of metastatic disease, particularly when located in the middle mediastinum.

7. Patients with contrast medium–enhancing lesions in the superior mediastinum who do not have symptoms are evaluated with an iodine-131 (^{131}I) scan. In a patient who does not have symptoms but has a positive scan indicative of a thyroid lesion and no identifiable active thyroid tissue elsewhere, careful observation without excision using serial CT scans to evaluate for growth is indicated.

8. Increased success has been reported in making a cytologic diagnosis preoperatively by using fine-needle aspiration (FNA) biopsy techniques (18-22 gauge needles). CT, echocardiography, endoscopic ultrasound and endobronchial ultrasound, because of better localization of the mass and improved placement of the needle, have increased the sensitivity of the technique. [15] Although a cytologic diagnosis of benign or malignant differentiation between masses can be made in about 90% of patients using FNA, a precise histologic diagnosis is not always possible. Obtaining core biopsy specimens using

cutting needles increases the accuracy of the precise histologic diagnosis and differentiation between benign and malignant lesions. Core biopsy techniques are particularly useful in the diagnosis of lymphomas, thymomas, and neural tumors.   Recent   advances   in immunohistochemical   and   core   biopsy techniques have allowed them to become more accurate for establishing the initial diagnosis of lymphoma, but it is probably better utilized for confirming recurrent disease.[17] .

Poorly   differentiated   malignant   tumors   of   the anterosuperior mediastinum, particularly thymomas, lymphomas,   germ   cell   tumors,   and   primary carcinomas, can have remarkably similar cytologic and morphologic appearances. In addition to light microscopy   using   special   staining   techniques, immunostaining techniques and electron microscopy of multiple sections of the tumor may be necessary to establish an accurate diagnosis,as shown in Table (4).

Table (4): Ultrastructural Characteristics of Mediastinal Tumors

TUMORS	ULTRASTRUCTURE

Carcinoid	Dense core granules, fewer monofilaments and desmosomes
Lymphoma	Absence of junctional attachments and epithelial features
Thymoma	Well-formed desmosome, bundles of tonofilaments
Germ cell	Prominent nucleoli, even chromatin, scant desmosomes, rare tonofilaments
Neuroblastoma	Neurosecretory granules, synaptic endings

9. When needle biopsy techniques are contraindicated or do not produce sufficient tissue for the histologic diagnosis,more invasive procedures are often required, such as mediastinoscopy, mediastinotomy, thoracoscopy, thoracotomy, or median sternotomy. Mediastinoscopy is a useful technique to evaluate and biopsy lesions of the middle mediastinum. This technique is often used to evaluate associated lymphadenopathy in this region. Biopsy of lesions in the anterosuperior mediastinum is best done using a limited anterior second or third interspace parasternal mediastinotomy or by thoracoscopy, which provides excellent exposure. Biopsies of posterior mediastinal masses may be approached thoracoscopically or through a limited posterolateral thoracotomy. A representative

section of the tissue obtained is submitted for immediate frozen-section analysis to establish adequacy of the biopsy before closing. Importantly, the incision is not made in the portals for potential radiation therapy. Lesions that appear resectable are excised. Median sternotomy provides optimal exposure for lesions in the anterosuperior mediastinum[18]. A transcervical approach using sternal elevators has been successfully used to resect tumors in the superior aspect of the anterosuperior mediastinum. Occasionally for extensive tumors of the anterosuperior mediastinum, a trans-sternal bilateral thoracotomy (clam shell) incision is indicated. Middle and posterior mediastinal masses are usually best excised through a posterolateral thoracotomy. Thoracoscopic and thoracoscopically assisted procedures are being used in diagnosing and treating a variety of mediastinal lesions in carefully selected patients. Although most patients undergo surgical procedures safely, patients with large anterosuperior or middle mediastinal masses, particularly children, have an increased risk for severe cardiorespiratory complications during general anesthesia. Patients with posture-related dyspnea and superior vena caval syndrome are at increased risk, and attempts to obtain a histologic diagnosis are limited to needle biopsies or open procedures done with local anesthesia. If a general anesthesia is required and there is concern about airway obstruction, an awake fiberoptic intubation is performed, rigid bronchoscopy available, and, if at all possible, anesthesia provided with inhalational agents only; muscle paralysis needs to be avoided in lesion of the tracheobronchial tree; Pancoast's syndrome; and Horner's syndrome resulting from involvement of the brachial and the cervical sympathetic chain. Symptoms may be systemic and related to production of neurohormonal agents.

1.9 Anterior and Superior Mediastinum

The common tumors in order of decreasing frequency are lymphomas, teratomas germ cell tumors, lymphangioma (cystic hygromas), and thymic tumors. Malignant lymphomas present most frequently in older children, and sometimes, diagnosis can be sought from non mediastinal areas such as bone marrow and nodal tissues. Among Non-Hodgkin lymphomas, the lymphoblastic subtype is most likely to present in the mediastinum. This is a diffuse, fast-growing tumor of T cell and
pre-B cell origin. Teratomas are the second most common tumors of the anterior mediastinum. They are derived from multiple germ cell layers and can have both cystic and solid
components. Teratomas frequently have calcifications, and only 25% of teratomas are malignant in pediatric

patients. β-HCG and a-fetoprotein can also help to differentiate various germ cell tumors and are especially important postoperatively as an early marker of recurrence. Seminomatous germ cell tumors are responsive to radiation therapy and should be distinguished from other types. Thymic cysts are usually asymptomatic but can become infected. Large lesions produce symptoms due to mass effect. Thymolipoma is benign, but along with thymic cysts, resection is indicated for proper diagnosis and prevention of complications. Thymomas originating in the thymic epithelium are usually aggressive, but account for less than 1% of mediastinal tumors. Thymoma associated with myasthenia gravis may produce autoantibodies to acetylcholine receptors which leads to progressive muscle weakness. Resection produces some improvement in symptoms for 30-50% of these children[19].

1.10   Middle Mediastinum

Pericardial cysts are benign, fluid-containing cysts lined with mesothelium. They are usually asymptomatic and CT imaging can provide accurate diagnosis. When the diagnosis is uncertain or the cysts become too large, thoracotomy or thoracoscopic resection or evacuation of the cysts should be performed. Pericardial effusion may, on rare occasions, represent underlying pathology such as cardiac hemangioma or rhabdomyoma. Bronchogenic cysts develop from abnormal budding of the tracheal diverticulum or ventral portion of the foregut. These mucus filled cysts are lined with bronchial epithelium and are frequently located at paraesophageal, paratracheal, or perihilar regions. Excision is performed electively to avoid the complications of infection, hemorrhage, or problems due to mass effects. Complete resection via thoracotomy or video-assisted thorocoscopy is the preferred treatment of bronchogenic cysts; recurrence and malignancy are extremely rare[20].

1.11 Posterior Mediastinum

The posterior mediastinum is the common site of benign and malignant neurogenic tumors. Sixty percent are malignant, most often neuroblastoma or ganglioneuroblastoma, and thirty percent are benign tumors such as ganglioneuroma, neurofibroma or schwannoma. The remaining 10% represent miscellaneous mesenchymal tumors or granulomas. Enteric duplication cysts may occur in this location, are lined by esophageal or gastric epithelium, and occasionally communicate with a viscus lumen. Most are asymptomatic and benign. Treatment is usually complete resection, but stripping of the mucosal lining of a foregut duplication may be adequate for long tubular duplications. Neuroenteric cysts are foregut duplications that also have connections to the spinal canal. They often present as an intraspinal mass. MRI

or CT with myelogram should be considered when a posterior mediastinal
mass is associated with vertebral anomalies. Total excision is recommended with simultaneous laminectomy as necessary[12].

1.12 Treatment

In general, the surgical approach to mediastinal masses depends on location, size and pathology. Thoracoscopy can be useful for resection or biopsy in approachable lesions, such as foregut duplications (enteric cysts and duplications, bronchogenic cysts, neurenteric cysts) and simple solid masses. Large anterior mediastinal masses are best approached through a median sternotomy[19]. For cysts, regardless of symptoms, removal should be seriously considered to prevent future complications of infection, bleeding or compression on adjacent normal structures. For similar reasons, benign mediastinal tumors should also be resected. Ganglioneuromas and neurofibromas often remain encapsulated and can be easily removed. The role of surgery regarding malignant tumors spans the spectrum from diagnostic procedures to complete resection or debulking of the tumor mass to relieve complications. Patients with Non-Hodgkin's lymphoma and bulky anterior mediastinal involvement may require surgical intervention for respiratory symptoms, pleural effusion or superior vena cava syndrome. Neuroblastomas, when found in early stages (I or II), are considered for complete primary resection. Seminomatous tumors are treated with chemotherapy and radiation, while germ cell tumors of other origin are treated with resection or debulking followed by chemotherapy[19].

1.13 Outcome

Prognosis depends on the underlying pathology. Patients with benign cysts and tumors have excellent outcomes with complete recovery. Recent protocols for Hodgkin's disease have improved the overall 5-year survival, which is now approaching 90%. Although, the youngest patients have the best prognosis, overall prognosis for Neuroblastoma remains poor[21].

Chapter two

Aim of study:

1. 1Mediastinal tumors in children comprise a heterogeneous group of lesions that have a range of embryonic origins. They may present as benign cysts, as well as malignant lesions.
2. To describe the diagnostic procedures, the treatments and outcomes of a group of children and adolescents with mediastinal tumors.

Patients and Methods:

1. This is a retrospective analysis of (35) children with mediastinal tumors who were treated at medical city Thoracic and Vascular surgery department , from January 2009 to December 2010. All patients were submitted to some kind

       of surgical procedure: diagnostic, therapeutic, or both.

2. Information about patients included in this study were retrieved from patients hospital records, adults beyond 16 years of age were excluded. Demographic data of patients were reviewed. The study included site of tumors, diagnostic aids, and management of patients.

Chapter three
<u>Results</u>

Thirty five patients with pediatrics primary mediastinal masses were identified. There were 6 females (19%) and 29 males (81%) in this study (M/F=4/1). The patients' ages ranged from 14 days to 15 years at the time of diagnosis with a mean age of 8 years and 4 months. Seven patients (20%) were asymptomatic and 21 patients (60%) had respiratory symptoms (cough, strider, Dyspnea), and the other seven patients (20%) had fever and fatigue. Most of patients in this study were referred from Al-Iskan Pediatric Hospital or Pediatrics Hospital in Medical City. All patients were submitted to complete investigations like CXR, CT scan and standard hematological and biochemical investigations.

Operations were done in all patients as follows: 19 patients had thoractomy (7 right and 12 left thoractomy).

6 patients had lymph node biopsy (supraclavicular) and ten patients with mediastinotomy. (Digram1)

Diagram 1: types of surgery

The mediastinal localization of the tumors is given in (Fig.6). For the whole series, 13 patients (37%) had tumors in the anterior mediastinum. In this study, of these tumors, Lymphoma were the most common masses, representing more than half (7/13) of cases. There were 15 tumors (43%) in the middle mediastinum. These consisted primarily of lymphomas and cardiac tumors. In the posterior

Table 4

mediastinum, there were seven tumors (20%), the most common of which was neurogenic tumors (Table 4 and Fig.6)

Histology(n)	NO.	0–1 year	2–5 years years	6–10 years	11–15 years
Lymphoma	16	-	1	5	10
Neurogenic tumors	6	1	3	1	1
Cystic lesions	5	-	1	1	3
Thymic pathologies	2	2	-	-	
Germ cell tumors	5	-	1	2	2
Cardiac epithelioid	1	1	-	-	-

Fig 6: types and localization of mediastinal tumors

	Lymphoma	Neurogenic tumors 2	Cystic lesions 3	Germ cell tumors 4	Cardiac epithelioid	Thymic pathologies
	7			3	1	2
...dle 2	9		4	2		
Posterior 3		6	1			

Histology results were variable (Table 5). 16 patients had lymphoma; of which 11 were Hodgkin's and 5 were lymphoblastic disease. Six patients had neurogenic tumors of which 4 Neurofibroma, one neuroblastoma, and one Meningocele. Five patients had cystic lesion all of them were bronchogenic cyst. Two patients had thymic hyperplasia. Five patients with germ cell tumors out of which three teratoma and two were seminoma. There was also one patient with a cardiac tumor (2.8%) the histological examination of which shows angiomyolipoma. Lymphomas were the most common tumors (N=16) and represented 46% of our patients . They generally presented in the teen years and were located in the middle mediastinum. Lymphomas were Hodgkin's disease in 11 patients (70%) and non- Hodgkin's lymphoma in the remaining 5 patients . Neurogenic tumors represented 17.2% of our total group and were the second most common mediastinal tumor

The thymic pathologies were seldom and represented 5.7% of the total group (2/35). All thymic lesions were resected without complication.

Table 5: Tumor Histology

Histopathology	NO.	Subdivision
Lymphoma	16	Hodgkin's (11) - Lymphoblastic (5)
Neurogenic	6	Neurofibroma (4) - Neuroblastoma (1) –Meningocele (1)

Cystic	5	Bronchogenic cyst (5)
Thymic	2	hyperplasia (2)
Germ cell	5	Teratoma (3)- seminoma (2)
Cardiac	1	Angiomyolipoma

Fig.7 : mediastinal tumor age incidence

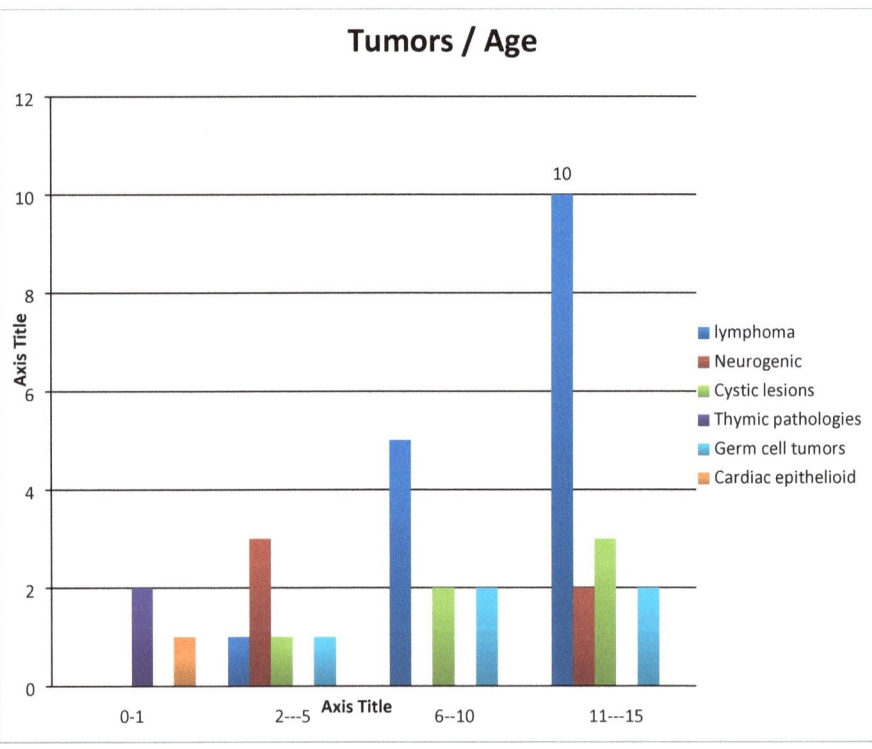

Mortality only two cases out of 35 (5.7)% one case 14 days myocardial mass multiple punch biopsies done patient admitted ICU death day two , second case is posterior mass which is Meningocele combined surgery with neurosurgery complete evacuation and Dura repaired day five discharge after five days die at home meningitis ?

Chapter four

Discussion

The most important factors in the management of an infant or child with a mediastinal mass are the nature of the disease, age, presenting symptoms and location of the mass on X-ray. The symptomatology of a primary mediastinal tumor may vary from patient to patient and usually depends on its anatomic location, size and nature. In our experience, a significant proportion of patients were symptomatic (80%) when first seen, with respiratory problems being the most common symptoms, consistent with other reports in The Turkish Journal of Pediatrics 2006[23] . Physical signs related to mediastinal tumors have not been well defined and our patients were usually free of gross abnormality. All patients in this study underwent complete physical examination, biochemical analysis and chest radiography as an initial investigation Developments in the diagnostic modalities have changed the approach of this initial workup. In our study, the introduction of computed tomography (CT) increased percentage of patients studied by CT. The patients with a mass located in the posterior mediastinum were also evaluated by magnetic resonance imaging (MRI). In such patients, the level of urinary VMA during the initial diagnostic evaluation was not done in our study. We did not perform a transthoracic fine needle aspiration biopsy; however, video-assisted thoracoscopic surgery, and/or cervical mediastinoscopy were the procedures not used in our study but Turkish[23] study of Pediatrics 2006 used in some patients to reach a definitive diagnosis . Our most common tumor was also lymphoma, which is consistent with literature. Our patients with lymphoma represented 45.7% of patients and received only chemotherapy and/or radiation therapy while in Turkish study represent 27% . Many studies have reported that neurogenic malignancies are the second most common pediatric mediastinal tumors1. Although neuroblastoma has been reported to be the most common neurogenic tumor in the pediatric population and occurs in children two years of age or younger, Neurofibroma was more common in our study. In our study, there were five germ cell tumors representing 14.2% of our patients. The incidence of germ cell tumors in this series was higher than previously reported Turkish study. In the pediatric age group, the frequency of benign thymic pathologies including thymic cysts and hyperplasia is usually more than in our population[22]. The two patients with thymic pathologies were successfully treated surgically through a right thoractomy. , the incidence of malignancy was 54.%. The patients having a tumor with benign histopathology (16/35) underwent a complete surgical resection and were discharged from the hospital in a good clinical condition except one patient with Meningocele were died after surgery on day five . They are still alive without evidence of recurrent disease. In all patients with lymphoma, surgery was not a part of treatment and they received medical and radiation therapy after discharge while in Turkish study only five . The surgical approach to these tumors has changed significantly over time. In the past, death was usually related either to the mass effect of the tumor or the complications of general anesthesia, but with refinements in surgical technique and anesthetic management, the mortality rate significantly decreased following surgical intervention. The significant increase in median sternotomy possibly reflects the increased experience of cardiothoracic surgeons with this incision. and anterior mediastonomy as the surgical and/or diagnostic procedure has greatly increased as well. . In conclusion, primary pediatric mediastinal malignancies are relatively common in infants and children. Lymphoma, neurogenic tumors and cystic lesions predominated. With improved surgical techniques and therapeutic regimens, the primary pediatric mediastinal tumors can be treated with acceptable morbidity and mortality rates. The differences between the age groups should also be considered when dealing with a mediastinal mass.

Conclusion:

- Mediastinal tumors in children and adolescents represent an important cause of morbidity/mortality.

- The most common tumors at the anterior mediastinum were lymphomas.

- posterior mediastinum the most common were neurogenic tumors.

- Surgery is an important step for the diagnosis and treatment of such lesions.

- The patients with a mass located in the posterior mediastinum were also evaluated by magnetic resonance imaging (MRI). In such patients, the level of urinary VMA during the initial diagnostic evaluation

- In all patients with lymphoma, surgery was not a part of treatment and they received medical and radiation therapy after discharge

- video-assisted thoracoscopic surgery, and/or cervical mediastinoscopy

Chapter five
Reference

1. Davis RD, Oldham HN, Sabiston DC: Primary cysts and neoplasms of the mediastinum: Recent changes in clinical presentation, methods of diagnosis, management, and results. Ann Thorac Surg 1987; 44:229-237.

2. Churchill Livingstone, 1995 Mediastinum : In Gray's Anatomy: The Anatomical Basis of Medicine and Surgery, 38th ed.. New York,

3. Shields TW: The mediastinum, its compartments and the mediastinal lymph nodes. General Thoracic Surgery,, 5th ed..
Philadelphia, Lippincott Williams & Wilkins, 2000

4. http://info.med.yale.edu/surgery/anatomy/graphics/unrestricted/grays/jpg/chapter3/F66124-003-f086.jpg

5. Colice GL, Shafazand S, Griffin JP, et al: Physiologic evaluation of the patient with lung cancer being considered for resectional surgery: ACCP evidenced-based clinical practice guidelines (2nd edition). *Chest* 132(3 Suppl):161S, 2007.

6. Philippart Al, Farmer DL. Benign mediastinal cysts and tumors. In: Oneill JA, Jr .,Rowe MI, Grosfeld JL et al, eds. Pediatric Surgery, ed 5, St. Louis: Mosby 1998.

7. Grosfeld JL, Skinner MA, Rescorla FJ et al. Mediastinal tumors in children: Experience with 196 cases. Ann Surg Oncol 1994; 1(2):121-127.

8. Yolonda L. Colson, MD, PhD Chapter 131, Overview—Mediastinal Diseases, Benign or Malignant

9. Pediatric Surgery, Robert M. Arensman, Daniel A. P. Stephen Almond.©2000 Landes bioscience Overview—Mediastinal Diseases, Benign or Malignant

10. Panelli F, Erickson RA, Prasad VM: Evaluation of mediastinal masses by endoscopic ultrasound and endoscopic ultrasound-guided fine needle aspiration. *Am J Gastroenterol* 2001; 96:401-408.

11. Christine L. Lau, MD Michigan Sabiston & Spencer Surgery of the Chest, 7th ed., Copyright © 2005 Saunders, An Imprint of Elsevier The Mediastinum

12. Saenz NC, Schnitzer JJ, Eraklis AE et al. Posterior mediastinal masses. J Pediatr Surg 1993; 28(2):172-176.

13. Nakata H, Egashira K, Watanabe H, et al: MRI of bronchogenic cysts. J Comput Assist Tomogr 1993; 17:267-270

14. Kostakoglu L, Leonard JP, Kuji I, et al: Comparison of fluorine-18 fluorodeoxyglucose positron emission tomography and Ga-67 scintigraphy in evaluation of lymphoma. Cancer 2002; 94:879-888.

15.   Morgenthaler TI, Brown LR, Colby TV, et al: Thymoma. Mayo Clin Proc 1993; 68:110-1123

16.   Yanik GA, Levine JE, Matthay KK, et al: Pilot study of iodine-131-metaiodobenzylguanidine in combination with myeloablative chemotherapy and autologous stem-cell support for the treatment of neuroblastoma. *J Clin Oncol* 2002; 20:2142-2149.

17.   Brodeur GM, Pritchard J, Berthold F, et al: Revisions of the international criteria for neuroblastoma diagnosis, staging, and response to treatment [comment]. J Clin Oncol 1993; 11:1466-1477.

18.   Khoo K, Ho K, Nilsson B, et al: EUS-guided FNA immediately after unrevealing transbronchial needle aspiration in the evaluation of mediastinal lymphadenopathy: A prospective study. Gastrointest Endosc 2006; 63:215-220.

19.   Kern JA, Daniel TM, Tribble CG et al. Thorascopic diagnosis and treatment of mediastinal masses. Ann Thorac Surg 1993; 56(1):92-96.

20.   Robie DK, Gursoy MH, Pokorny WJ. Mediastinal tumors-airway obstruction and management. Semin Pediatr Surg 1994; 3(4):259-266.

21.   Turkish Journal of Pediatrics 2006; 48: 8-12 Original Childhood mediastinal masses in

infants and children Türkan Tansel[1], Ertan Onursal[1], Enver Dayıoğlu[1], Murat Başaran[1], Zerrin Sungur[2]

22.	Emre	Çamcı[2],	Dilek	Yılmazbayhan[3], Rukiye Eker4, Türkan Ertuğrul4 Departments of [1]Cardiovascular	Surgery,	[2]Anesthesiology, [3]Pathology, and 4Pediatrics, Istanbul University Istanbul Faculty of Medicine, İstanbul, Turkey

www.ingramcontent.com/pod-product-compliance
Lightning Source LLC
Chambersburg PA
CBHW040925180526
45159CB00002BA/611